DEDICATION

This book is dedicated to my Lord and savior, Yeshuah and also to my mom, Mrs. Odo Beatrice.

CONTENTS

Introduction.. 5

I. Understanding the Challenges 7

II. Building a Foundation..................................... 10

III. Time-Efficient Workouts................................. 12

IV. Incorporating Fitness into Daily Routines................. 14

V. Stress Management Techniques........................... 16

VI. Nutrition Tips for Busy Professionals.................... 18

VII. Overcoming Common Excuses........................... 20

VII. Balancing Work and Wellness............................ 22

IX. Conclusion... 24

FITNESS FOR BUSY PROFESSIONALS

HEALTH IS WEALTH AMONG PROFESSIONALS

CHUKWUMA KENNETH NNAEMEKA

Introduction:

In the relentless pace of the modern professional world, where deadlines loom large, and responsibilities are ever-expanding, the concept of personal well-being often finds itself relegated to the background. Yet, the very nature of the demanding professional lifestyle underscores the critical need for individuals to prioritize their health and fitness. Welcome to "Fitness for Busy Professionals," an eBook meticulously crafted to address the unique challenges faced by those navigating the fast-paced currents of contemporary careers.

1. The Modern Professional Lifestyle:

The unceasing demands of the modern professional lifestyle paint a vivid picture of fast-paced days, tight schedules, and the perpetual challenge of balancing personal and career responsibilities. This chapter delves into the intricacies of the daily grind, setting the stage for understanding the unique obstacles that busy professionals encounter on their journey to optimal health.

2. The Importance of Fitness for Busy Individuals:

As the narrative unfolds, we explore the profound impact of fitness on the lives of busy professionals. Beyond the aesthetics of a fit physique, we delve into the cognitive enhancements, stress resilience, and heightened productivity that result from a commitment to regular exercise. Discover how fitness isn't merely a luxury but a strategic imperative for navigating the rigors of a demanding professional life.

3. Setting Realistic Fitness Goals:

In a world that often feels like a perpetual race against time, setting realistic fitness goals becomes paramount. This chapter lays the foundation for a transformative journey by guiding busy professionals through the process of creating goals that are not only achievable but also tailored to the unique constraints of their schedules.

As we progress through the ensuing chapters, we will explore the multifaceted challenges faced by busy professionals, including time constraints, stress management, and maintaining a balanced nutrition plan. From building a solid fitness foundation to incorporating time-efficient workouts and stress management techniques, each section offers practical insights, actionable strategies, and tangible solutions for those seeking to infuse fitness into their daily routines.

Embark on this journey with us—a journey that goes beyond the gym, beyond conventional fitness advice, and is tailored specifically for individuals leading the charge in the dynamic realm of professional life. Let "Fitness for Busy Professionals" be your guide to reclaiming control over your well-being, enhancing your performance, and ultimately achieving a harmonious balance between career success and personal health.

Chapter 1: Understanding the Challenges

In the dynamic landscape of a busy professional's life, recognizing and comprehending the hurdles that impede the journey to fitness is the crucial first step. This chapter delves into the multifaceted challenges faced by busy professionals, offering insights and actionable strategies to overcome these obstacles and pave the way for a healthier, more balanced lifestyle.

Time Constraints

1. Analyzing Daily Schedules:

The cornerstone of effective time management lies in a deep understanding of our daily schedules. In this section, we'll dissect the typical day of busy professional, identifying pockets of time that can be optimized for fitness activities. From early morning routines to post-work rituals, we'll explore how to carve out dedicated time for exercise within the existing framework of daily commitments.

2. Overcoming Time Barriers:

Time constraints often serve as a formidable barrier to consistent exercise. Here, we'll explore practical strategies to overcome these barriers. From incorporating time-efficient workouts to leveraging technology for quick fitness sessions, we'll unravel innovative approaches that empower busy professionals to prioritize their well-being without compromising on their professional responsibilities.

Stress Management

1. Impact of Stress on Health:

Stress is an omnipresent companion in the world of professionals, but understanding its profound impact on health is pivotal. This section sheds light on the physiological and psychological consequences of chronic stress. Drawing connections between stress and various health issues, we emphasize the urgency of adopting stress management techniques as a foundational aspect of overall well-being.

2. Incorporating Fitness for Stress Relief:

Fitness serves as a potent antidote to the stresses of professional life. Here, we explore the symbiotic relationship between physical activity and stress relief. From the release of endorphins to the meditative benefits of certain exercises, busy professionals will discover how integrating fitness into their routines becomes a proactive strategy for managing stress and enhancing resilience.

Nutrition in a Busy World

1. Quick and Healthy Eating Habits:

In the hustle and bustle of professional life, maintaining a healthy diet can be challenging. This section provides practical tips for cultivating quick and healthy eating habits. From smart food choices to time-saving meal prep strategies, busy professionals will learn how to nourish their bodies efficiently without sacrificing nutritional quality.

2. Importance of Nutrient-Rich Foods:

Nutrition is the foundation of overall health and vitality. In this segment, we delve into the significance of nutrient-rich foods in sustaining energy levels and promoting optimal health. From highlighting key nutrients to exploring convenient sources of nutrition, busy professionals will gain valuable insights into fueling their bodies for peak performance.

As we navigate these challenges together, the aim is not only to recognize the hurdles but to equip busy professionals with practical tools and knowledge to overcome them. By understanding the unique time constraints, managing stress effectively, and embracing a nutrition plan tailored for a busy lifestyle, individuals will be better prepared to embark on a transformative fitness journey that seamlessly integrates with their professional commitments.

Chapter 2: Building a Foundation

In the pursuit of fitness amidst the demands of a busy professional life, establishing a robust foundation is paramount. This chapter is dedicated to guiding busy professionals through the process of self-assessment, identifying strengths and weaknesses, and creating realistic fitness plans tailored to the unique challenges they face. Let's delve into the essential elements that form the bedrock of a transformative fitness journey.

Assessing Current Fitness Levels

1. Fitness Assessments for Busy Professionals:

Understanding where you currently stand on your fitness journey is the first step towards progress. This section introduces practical fitness assessments specially designed for busy professionals. From assessing cardiovascular fitness to gauging strength and flexibility, these assessments provide a snapshot of your current physical condition, offering valuable insights to inform your fitness strategy.

2. Identifying Strengths and Weaknesses:

Every individual possesses unique strengths and faces specific challenges on their fitness journey. This segment explores how to discern these strengths and weaknesses through self-reflection and assessment results. Identifying areas of improvement becomes a powerful tool for crafting a targeted and effective fitness plan.

Creating Realistic Fitness Plans

1. Short, Effective Workouts:

Acknowledging time constraints, this section introduces the concept of short yet impactful workouts tailored for busy professionals. We'll explore time-efficient exercise routines that maximize results, incorporating a mix of cardiovascular exercises, strength training, and flexibility work. These workouts are designed to seamlessly integrate into your daily schedule, ensuring that fitness becomes an achievable and sustainable commitment.

2. Setting Achievable Milestones:

The journey to fitness is a series of incremental steps, and setting achievable milestones is crucial for sustained progress. This section outlines the process of establishing realistic short-term and long-term goals. Whether it's achieving a certain fitness level, completing a specific workout routine, or developing healthier habits, these milestones serve as guideposts, keeping you motivated and focused on your journey.

As you embark on the foundation-building phase of your fitness expedition, remember that progress is a personal and dynamic process. This chapter equips you with the tools to assess your starting point, identify areas for improvement, and set realistic goals that align with your busy professional life. In the chapters to come, we will delve deeper into time-efficient workouts and strategies for achieving these milestones, ensuring that your foundation is not just strong but resilient, setting the stage for a transformative and sustainable fitness journey.

Chapter 3: Time-Efficient Workouts

In the bustling world of busy professionals, time is a precious commodity. This chapter is dedicated to unraveling the power of time-efficient workouts tailored for the dynamic schedules of professionals on the go. Discover the transformative benefits of High-Intensity Interval Training (HIIT) and explore desk exercises designed to seamlessly integrate fitness into your daily routine.

High-Intensity Interval Training (HIIT)

1. Benefits for Busy Professionals:

High-Intensity Interval Training (HIIT) emerges as a beacon of efficiency in the realm of time-conscious workouts. This section outlines the specific benefits of HIIT for busy professionals. From enhanced calorie burn to improved cardiovascular health and increased metabolic rate, HIIT becomes a strategic ally in optimizing the impact of your workouts within limited time frames.

2. Sample HIIT Workouts:

Delve into the practical application of HIIT with a collection of sample workouts curated for busy professionals. These workouts are designed to be concise yet powerful, leveraging alternating intervals of intense exercise and brief rest periods. With routines customizable to your fitness level, these sample workouts provide a blueprint for incorporating HIIT seamlessly into your schedule, whether at home or in a gym.

Deskercise

1. Exercises for the Office:

Transform your workplace into a fitness-friendly environment with targeted desk exercises. This section introduces a repertoire of exercises that can be discreetly performed at your desk, requiring minimal space and no additional equipment. From seated stretches to desk squats, discover a range of movements that counteract the sedentary nature of office life, promoting flexibility, and alleviating tension.

2. Incorporating Movement into Daily Tasks:

Redefine the concept of multitasking by incorporating movement into your daily tasks. Learn how simple adjustments, such as taking the stairs, walking meetings, or brief stretching breaks, can contribute to your overall daily activity level. This section provides practical strategies for infusing movement seamlessly into your professional routine, ensuring that fitness becomes an integral part of your daily life.

As we explore the realm of time-efficient workouts, remember that the efficacy of these routines lies not just in their brevity but in their ability to deliver tangible results. Whether you're engaging in a quick HIIT session or discreetly incorporating desk exercises into your workday, these time-efficient workouts are crafted to align with the demands of your busy professional life. In the following chapters, we'll further explore strategies for incorporating fitness into your daily routines, ensuring that your journey to wellness remains not just effective but also sustainable.

Chapter 4: Incorporating Fitness into Daily Routines

In the perpetual motion of a busy professional's life, the integration of fitness into daily routines emerges as a key strategy for achieving sustainable well-being. This chapter explores innovative approaches to weave physical activity seamlessly into your day, from active commuting to micro-workouts that defy the constraints of time.

Active Commuting

1. Walking or Biking to Work:

Commuting provides a unique opportunity to infuse your daily routine with physical activity. Explore the benefits of opting for active modes of transportation, such as walking or biking to work. This section outlines the positive impacts on cardiovascular health, mental well-being, and overall energy levels. Discover practical tips for incorporating these active commuting options into your daily life, transforming the journey to and from work into an opportunity for fitness.

2. Making the Most of Commuting Time:

Uncover strategies to optimize your commuting time for fitness gains. Whether you're using public transportation or driving, learn how to leverage this time for activities that promote physical well-being. From mindfulness practices to simple stretches, this section provides creative ways to make the most of your daily commute, ensuring that even the busiest moments contribute to your overall fitness.

Micro-Workouts

1. Sneaking in Exercise throughout the Day:

Embrace the concept of micro-workouts—short, targeted bursts of exercise strategically sprinkled throughout your day. This section delves into the idea of breaking down traditional workout barriers, demonstrating how even the busiest professionals can sneak in moments of physical activity. Discover exercises that can be seamlessly integrated into your routine, transforming daily tasks into opportunities for movement.

2. Quick Exercise Breaks:

Explore the concept of quick exercise breaks as a means of recharging both your body and mind. This section offers a collection of brief yet effective exercises that can be performed during short breaks at work. From desk stretches to energizing movements, discover how these quick breaks can enhance focus, alleviate stress, and contribute to your overall fitness goals.

As we explore the integration of fitness into your daily routines, remember that small, consistent efforts can lead to significant and sustainable results. From transforming your commute into an active endeavor to embracing micro-workouts as part of your daily rhythm, these strategies are crafted to align seamlessly with the dynamic nature of your professional life. In the subsequent chapters, we'll delve into stress management techniques and nutritional tips tailored for the busy professional, ensuring a holistic approach to your wellness journey.

Chapter 5: Stress Management Techniques

In the fast-paced world of busy professionals, stress is an omnipresent companion. This chapter is dedicated to equipping you with effective stress management techniques, seamlessly integrating them into your daily routine. From the power of mindfulness to the symbiotic relationship between fitness and mental well-being, discover strategies that foster balance and resilience in the face of professional pressures.

Mindful Practices

1. Incorporating Mindfulness into Daily Life:

Delve into the transformative practice of mindfulness and learn how to infuse it into your daily life. This section explores practical ways to cultivate mindfulness amidst the whirlwind of professional responsibilities. From mindful breathing during meetings to incorporating awareness into routine tasks, discover how mindfulness becomes a potent tool for managing stress and enhancing overall well-being.

2. Stress-Relieving Breathing Exercises:

Uncover the calming influence of intentional breathing exercises. This segment introduces a variety of techniques designed to alleviate stress and promote a sense of calm. Whether it's deep diaphragmatic breathing or rhythmic breath cycles, these exercises can be seamlessly integrated into your day, providing an accessible means to manage stress and cultivate a more centered mindset.

Fitness and Mental Wellbeing

1. Connection between Exercise and Stress Reduction:

Explore the profound connection between physical exercise and stress reduction. This section delves into the physiological and psychological mechanisms through which exercise acts as a natural stress reliever. By understanding this connection, you'll be empowered to leverage your fitness routine as a strategic tool for mitigating stress and promoting mental well-being.

2. Mind-Body Practices for Balance:

Expand your approach to stress management with mind-body practices that harmonize mental and physical well-being. From yoga to tai chi, discover exercises that unite movement, breath, and mindfulness. This section outlines how incorporating mind-body practices into your fitness routine fosters balance, reduces stress, and promotes a holistic sense of wellness.

As you explore these stress management techniques, remember that the journey to balance is a dynamic and personalized process. From mindful practices that ground you in the present to the symbiotic relationship between fitness and mental well-being, these strategies are crafted to empower you in the face of professional demands. In the upcoming chapters, we'll delve into nutritional tips specifically tailored for busy professionals, completing the holistic framework for your wellness journey.

Chapter 6: Nutrition Tips for Busy Professionals

Fueling your body with the right nutrients is a cornerstone of holistic well-being, especially for busy professionals navigating demanding schedules. This chapter is dedicated to providing practical nutrition tips that align with the dynamic lifestyle of busy individuals, focusing on meal planning, smart snacking, hydration, and choosing energizing foods.

Planning Quick and Healthy Meals

1. Meal Prepping Strategies:

Dive into the world of meal prepping and discover efficient strategies tailored for busy professionals. This section outlines how dedicating a short time to plan and prepare meals in advance can streamline your nutrition. From batch cooking to creating versatile components, learn how meal prepping empowers you to make healthier choices even in the midst of a hectic schedule.

2. Smart Snacking Choices:

Snacking is an integral part of a busy professional's day, but it can also be an opportunity for mindful nutrition. Explore smart snacking choices that provide sustained energy and support your fitness goals. From nutrient-dense snacks to portion control strategies, this section guides you in making informed choices that keep you energized and focused throughout the day.

Hydration and Energy

1. Importance of Staying Hydrated:

Uncover the critical role hydration plays in maintaining optimal energy levels. This section emphasizes the importance of staying adequately hydrated for overall health and vitality. Practical tips for incorporating more water into your day, recognizing hydration cues, and choosing hydrating foods are explored to ensure you remain energized and focused in your professional endeavors.

2. Choosing Energizing Foods:

Explore a spectrum of energizing foods that fuel both body and mind. From complex carbohydrates for sustained energy to nutrient-rich foods that support cognitive function, this section provides insights into making wise food choices. Discover how to create balanced meals that enhance your productivity and contribute to your overall well-being.

As you embrace these nutrition tips, remember that nourishing your body is an essential component of your fitness journey. By planning quick and healthy meals, making smart snacking choices, prioritizing hydration, and selecting energizing foods, you're not only fueling your body but also optimizing your performance in your professional life. In the upcoming chapters, we'll delve into strategies for overcoming common excuses and maintaining a healthy work-life balance, completing the comprehensive guide to fitness for busy professionals.

Chapter 7: Overcoming Common Excuses

In the journey to fitness, excuses can often be formidable roadblocks. This chapter is dedicated to empowering busy professionals to identify and overcome common excuses that may hinder their commitment to a healthier lifestyle. Explore strategies to surmount these obstacles, foster accountability partnerships, and develop a resilient mindset that propels you toward your fitness goals.

Identifying Excuses and Obstacles

Excuses come in various forms, from lack of time to perceived barriers. This section encourages self-reflection to identify the excuses and obstacles that may be impeding your fitness journey. By acknowledging these challenges, you pave the way for targeted strategies to overcome them.

Strategies for Overcoming Fitness Barriers

1. Accountability Partnerships:

Discover the power of accountability partnerships in maintaining consistency on your fitness journey. This section outlines how aligning with a workout buddy or a support network can significantly enhance motivation and commitment. Learn how shared goals and mutual encouragement can transform the way you approach fitness, turning it into a collaborative and enjoyable endeavor.

2. Developing a Resilient Mindset:

Cultivate a resilient mindset that acts as a shield against common excuses. This segment explores mental strategies to overcome setbacks, manage stress, and stay committed to your fitness goals. By fostering a positive and resilient mindset, you'll navigate challenges with grace, turning obstacles into opportunities for growth.

As you delve into the strategies presented in this chapter, remember that overcoming excuses is a pivotal step toward creating lasting and positive change in your life. By identifying and addressing the common excuses that often surface in a busy professional's journey, and by embracing accountability partnerships and cultivating a resilient mindset, you are setting the stage for a transformative and sustainable approach to fitness. In the subsequent chapters, we'll explore strategies for balancing work and wellness, ensuring that your fitness journey is seamlessly integrated into your professional and personal life.

Chapter 8: Balancing Work and Wellness

Maintaining a harmonious equilibrium between work and wellness is a crucial aspect of a busy professional's journey to fitness. In this chapter, we explore strategies for creating a healthy work-life balance and prioritizing fitness within the intricate tapestry of professional responsibilities.

Creating a Healthy Work-Life Balance

Navigating the delicate balance between work and personal life is paramount for sustained well-being. This section delves into practical tips for creating a healthy work-life balance. From setting boundaries to time management strategies, discover how to carve out space for both professional success and personal wellness.

Strategies for Prioritizing Fitness

1. Scheduling Fitness Time:

Explore the art of intentional scheduling when it comes to fitness. This section provides insights into optimizing your calendar to make time for regular exercise. Discover how to treat your fitness commitments with the same level of importance as work obligations, ensuring that physical activity becomes an integral and non-negotiable part of your routine.

2. Integrating Wellness into Professional Goals:

Align your professional and wellness goals for a holistic approach to success. This segment outlines strategies for integrating wellness into your professional aspirations. By viewing fitness as an ally in achieving your career objectives, you'll create a synergistic relationship between work and wellness, fostering a sense of purpose and fulfillment. As you immerse yourself in the strategies outlined in this chapter, remember that the true essence of a successful and fulfilling life lies in the delicate dance between professional achievements and personal well-being. By creating a healthy work-life balance and implementing strategies to prioritize fitness within your professional framework, you're not only enhancing your physical health but also fortifying your resilience and capacity for sustained success. In the concluding chapter, we'll recap key strategies, provide encouragement for sustaining fitness habits, and empower busy professionals to prioritize their health for lasting well-being.

Chapter 9: Conclusion: Prioritizing Your Health

Congratulations on reaching the final chapter of "Fitness for Busy Professionals." This journey has been a comprehensive exploration of strategies designed to empower you to integrate fitness seamlessly into your dynamic professional life. As we conclude, let's reflect on key strategies, offer encouragement for sustaining fitness habits, and reinforce the profound importance of prioritizing your health.

Recap of Key Strategies

Throughout this eBook, we've navigated the intricacies of a busy professional's life, addressing challenges and providing practical solutions. Let's briefly recap key strategies:

Understanding the Challenges: Acknowledge the unique obstacles faced by busy professionals, from time constraints to stress management and nutrition in a fast-paced world.

Building a Foundation: Assess your current fitness levels, identify strengths and weaknesses, and create realistic fitness plans tailored to your busy schedule.

Time-Efficient Workouts: Embrace the efficiency of High-Intensity Interval Training (HIIT) and desk exercises to make the most of limited time.

Incorporating Fitness into Daily Routines: Seamlessly integrate fitness into your day through active commuting, micro-workouts, and strategic breaks.

Stress Management Techniques: Cultivate mindfulness, recognize the connection between fitness and mental well-being, and incorporate mind-body practices for balance.

Nutrition Tips for Busy Professionals: Plan quick and healthy meals, make smart snacking choices, stay hydrated, and choose energizing foods.

Overcoming Common Excuses: Identify and overcome excuses by fostering accountability partnerships and developing a resilient mindset.

Balancing Work and Wellness: Create a healthy work-life balance and prioritize fitness by scheduling dedicated time and integrating wellness into professional goals.

Encouragement for Sustainable Fitness Habits

Embarking on a fitness journey is a commitment to long-term well-being. Sustainable habits are not formed overnight, and progress is often gradual. Celebrate your achievements, no matter how small, and be patient with yourself during setbacks. Consistency is key, and every step you take towards prioritizing your health is a victory.

Empowering Busy Professionals to Prioritize Their Health

Your health is an invaluable asset, and prioritizing it is a strategic investment in your personal and professional success. As a busy professional, you are not exempt from the benefits of a healthy lifestyle; in fact, you stand to gain even more. A resilient body and a focused mind are indispensable tools in navigating the challenges of your career.

Empower yourself by recognizing that your well-being is not a luxury but a necessity. It is the foundation upon which you build your professional achievements and personal fulfillment. By integrating fitness into your routine, you're not just investing in physical health but also enhancing mental resilience, improving productivity, and fostering a positive mindset. Remember, the journey to optimal health is ongoing. Use the strategies provided in this eBook as stepping stones, adapting them to your evolving needs. Continuously assess your goals, celebrate your successes, and embrace the transformative power of a balanced and healthy lifestyle.

Thank you for joining me on this journey to prioritize your health as a busy professional. May your commitment to fitness become a catalyst for sustained well-being, and may you find enduring success both in your professional endeavors and in the vibrant tapestry of your life.

ABOUT THE AUTHUR

Chukwuma Kenneth Nnaemeka

Chukwuma Kenneth Nnaemeka is an expert in building construction and management. He studied Estate Management and Valuation and currently in third year studying Civil Engineering.

He is the CEO in Chuksman Construction and Development Company Limited.

What makes this book unique is that everything inside are from both detailed research and personal experience.

www.ingramcontent.com/pod-product-compliance
Lightning Source LLC
Chambersburg PA
CBHW060912260726
48661CB00008B/3597